RICKY Overcomes Fear

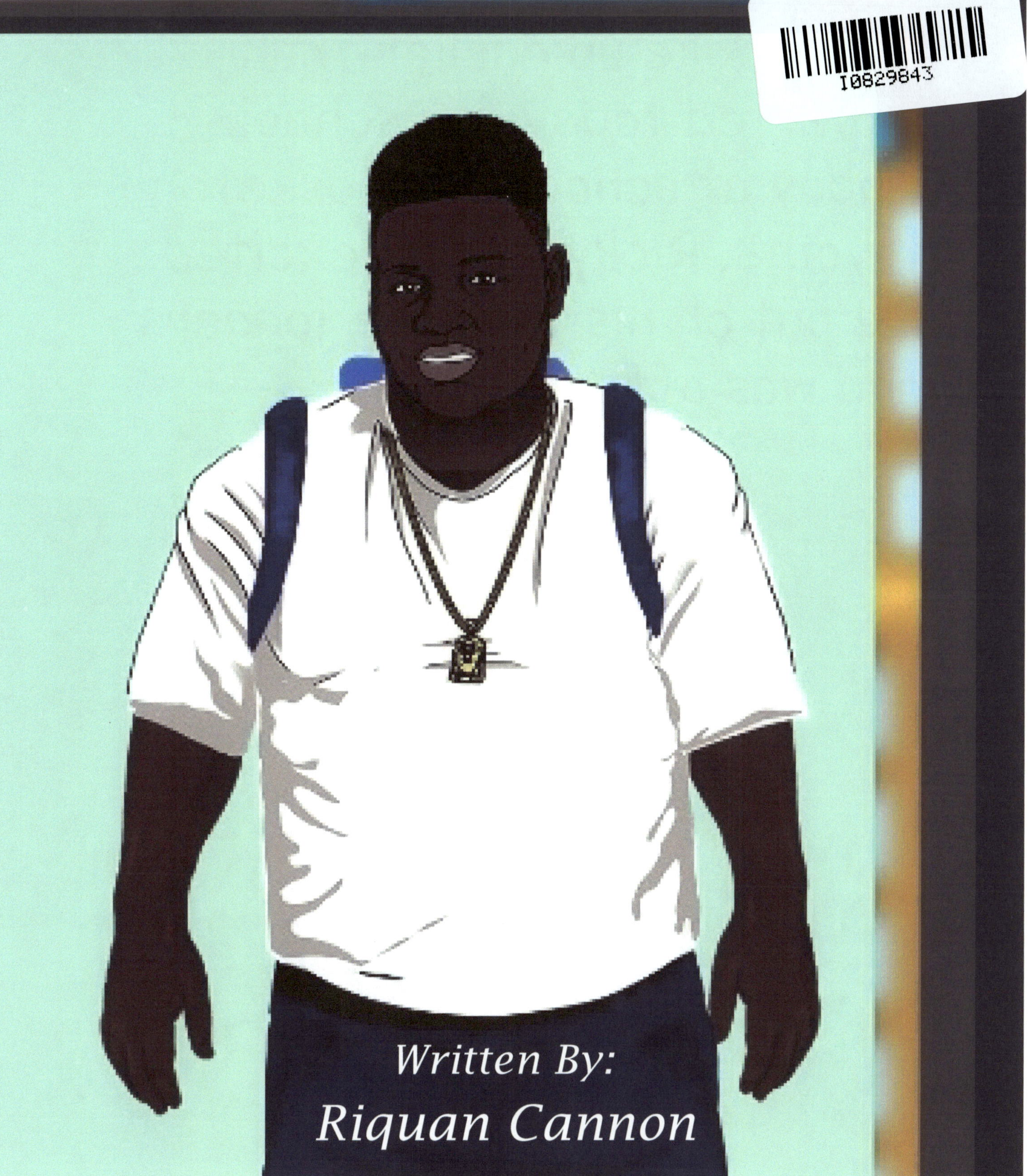

Written By:

Riquan Cannon

Ricky woke up earlier than expected today for school. Today at school was basketball tryouts. Ricky was so excited. He put on his favorite joggers and was off to school.

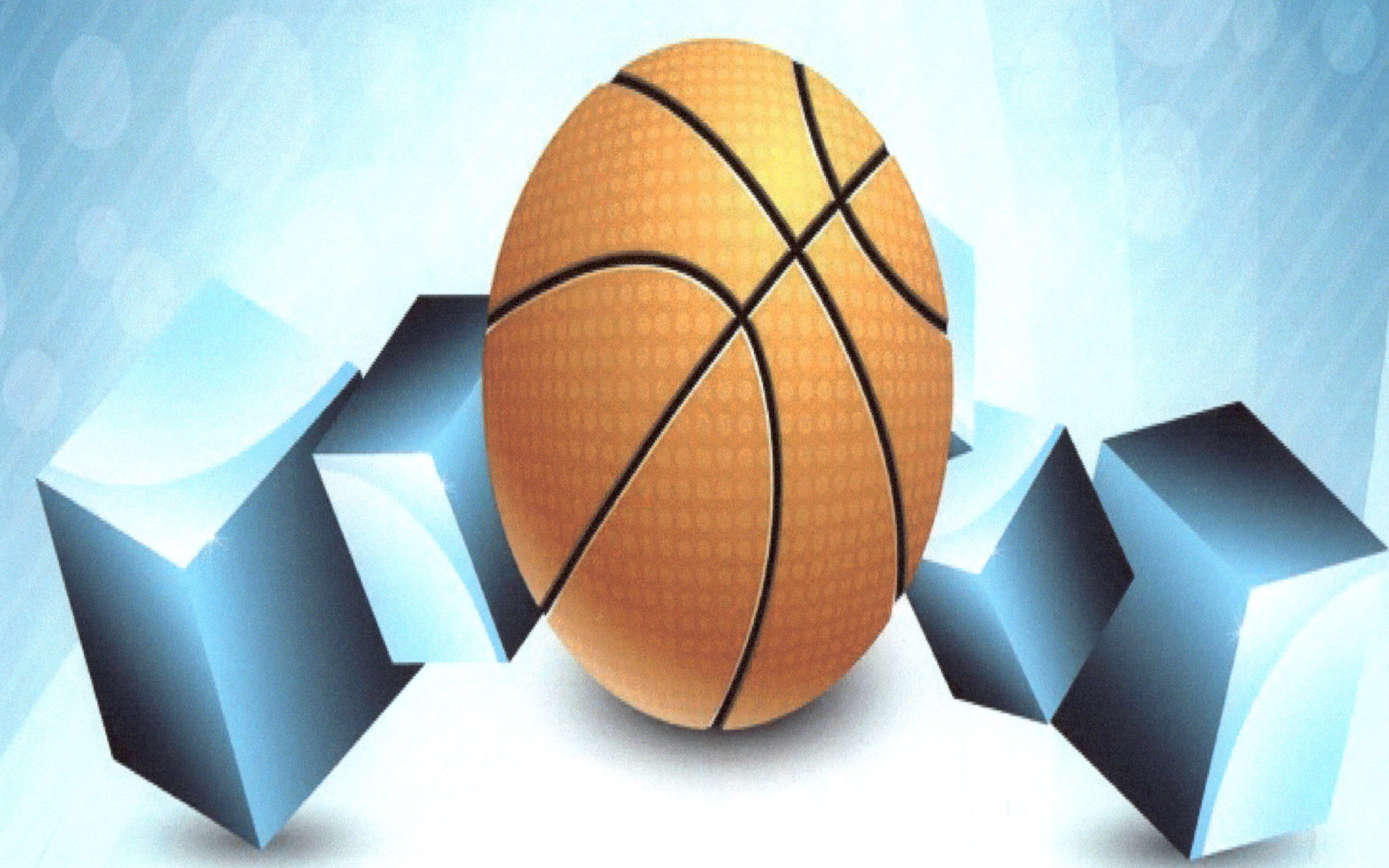

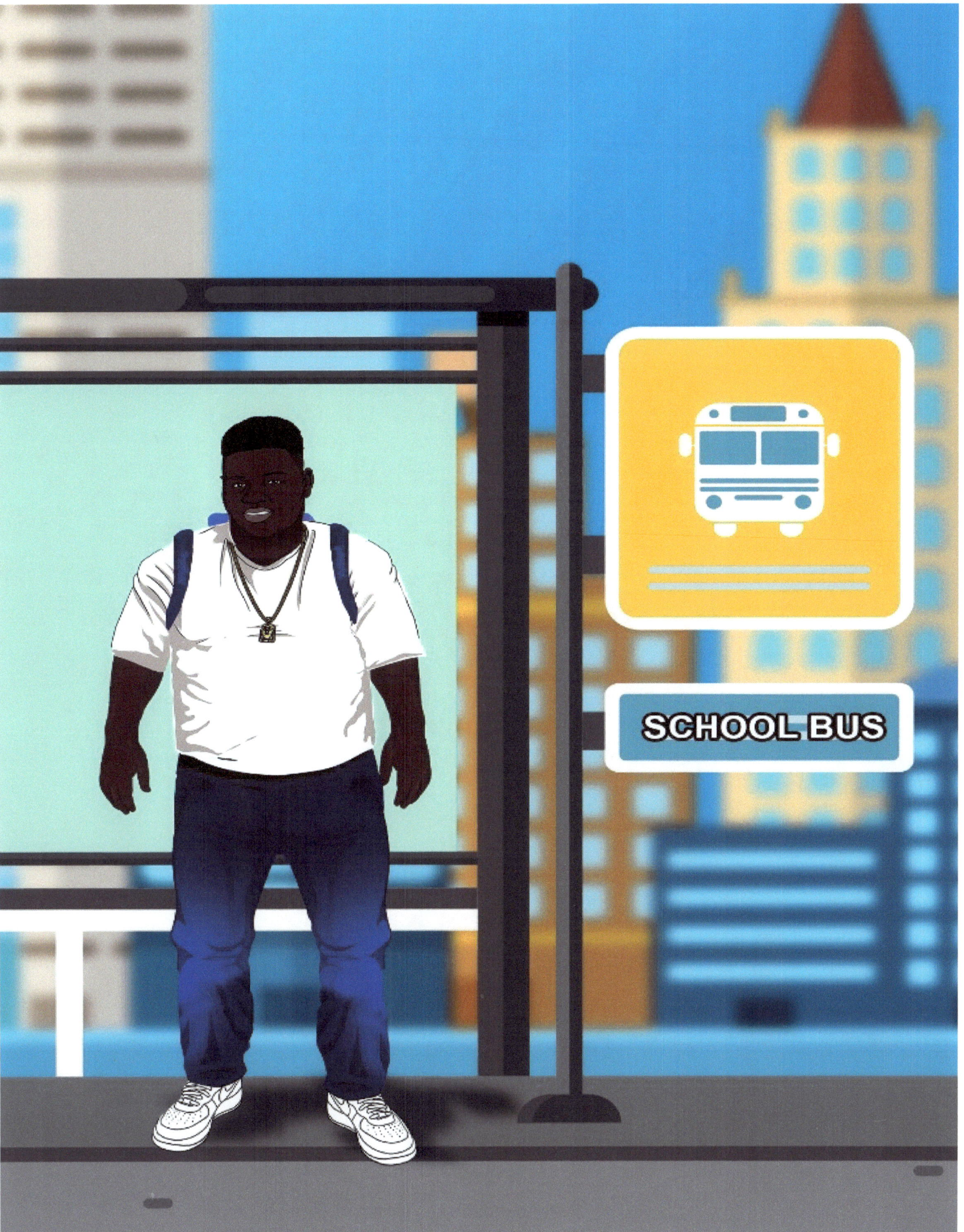
SCHOOL BUS

The day couldn't go by fast enough. Ricky anxiously waited until the bell rang at 2:25pm. Tick, Tock, Tick, Tock....Tick.... RINNNNNGGGGGG!!! Ricky jumped from his seat and rushed out of class to the gym. He signed in and took a seat.

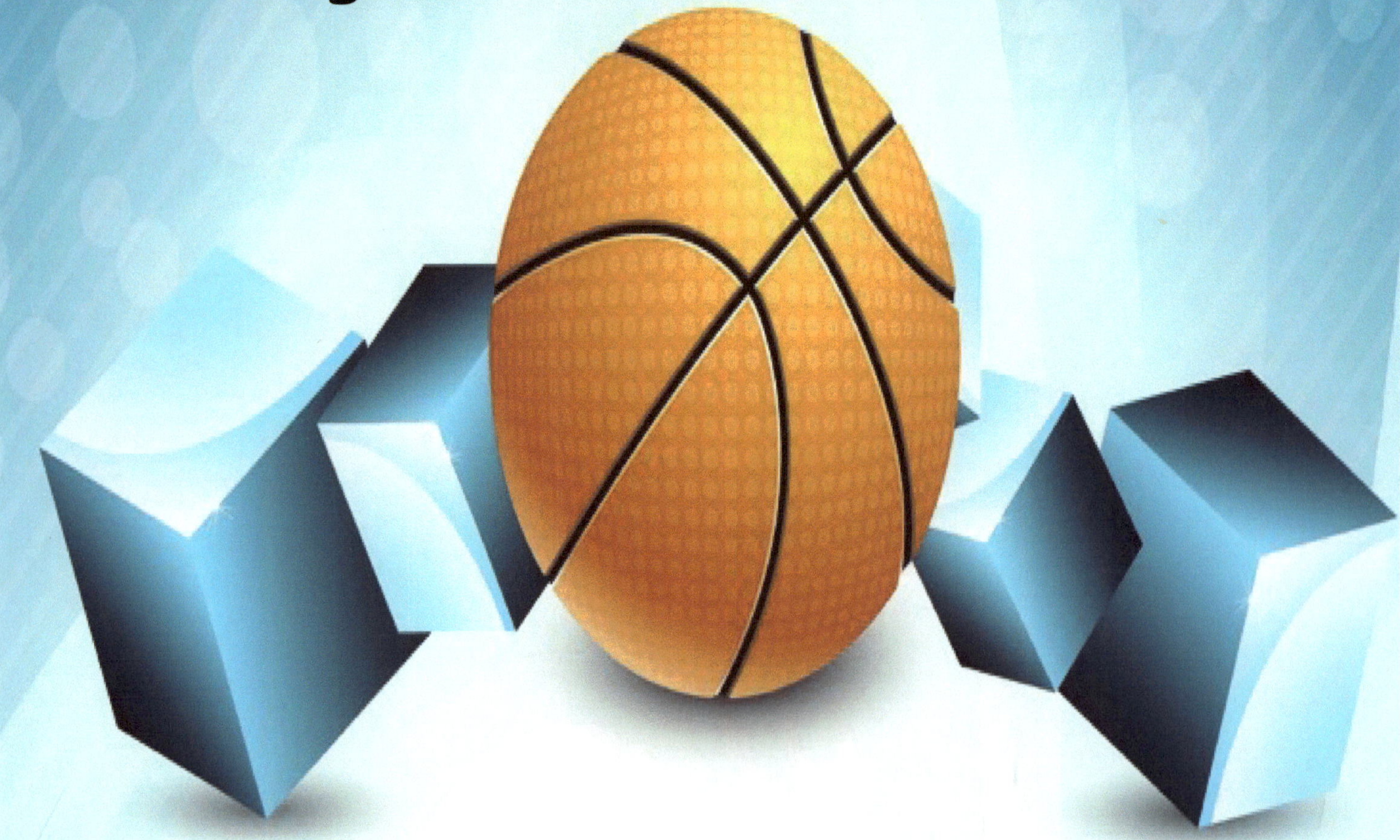

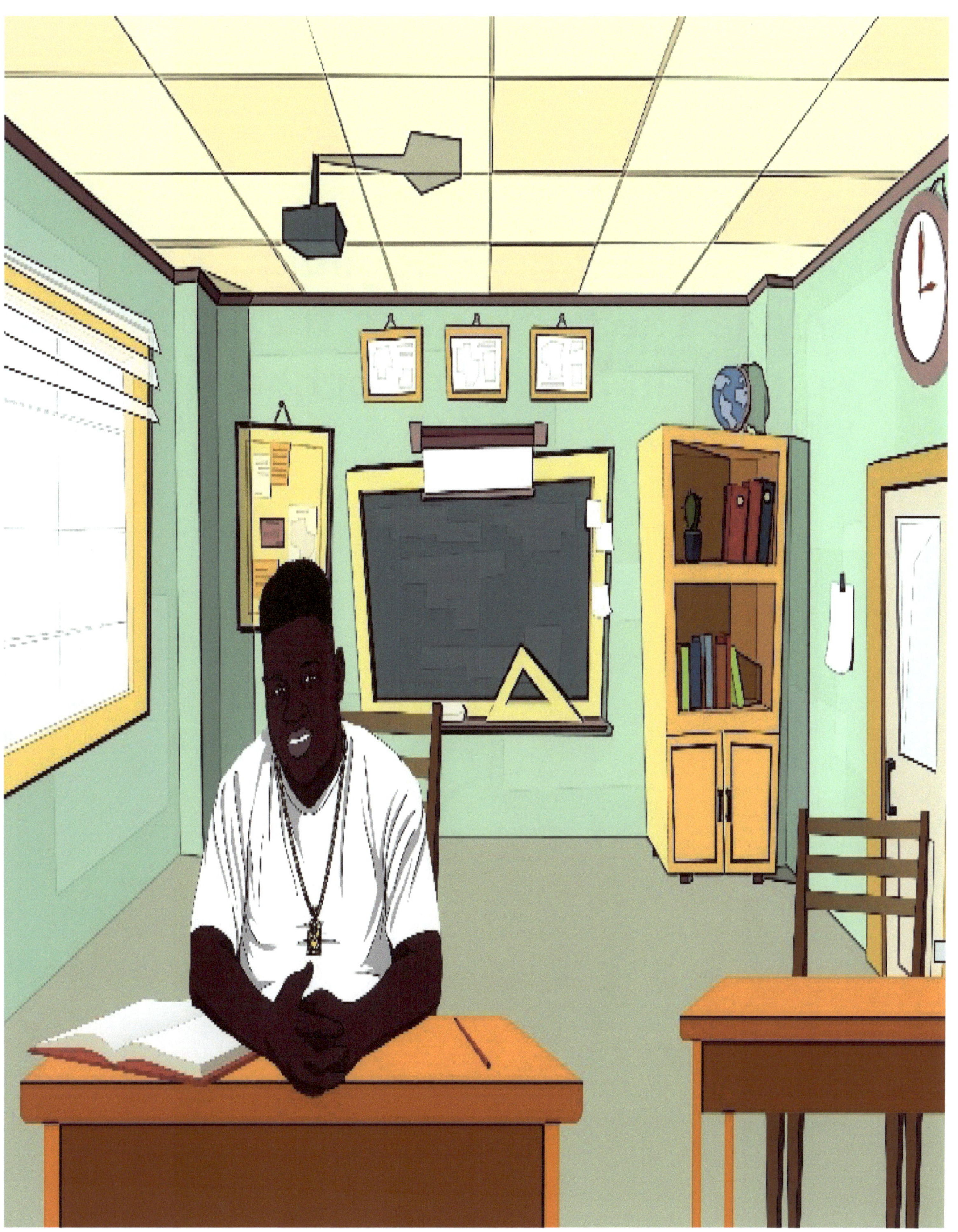

Ricky knew he was going to make the team he is the best player in his neighborhood.

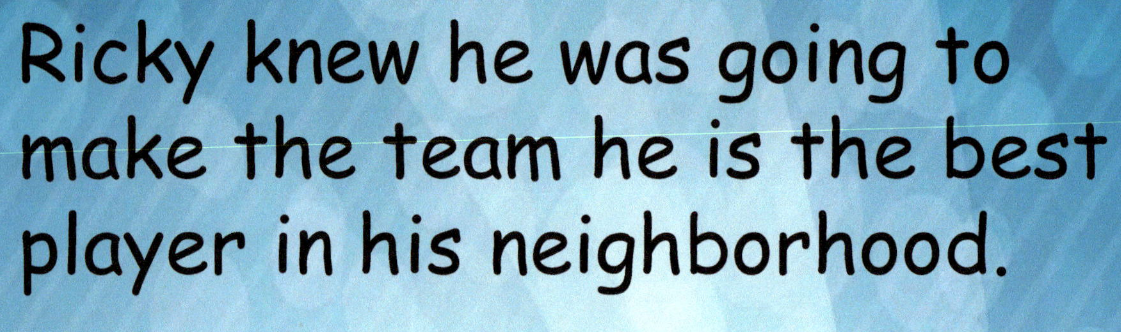

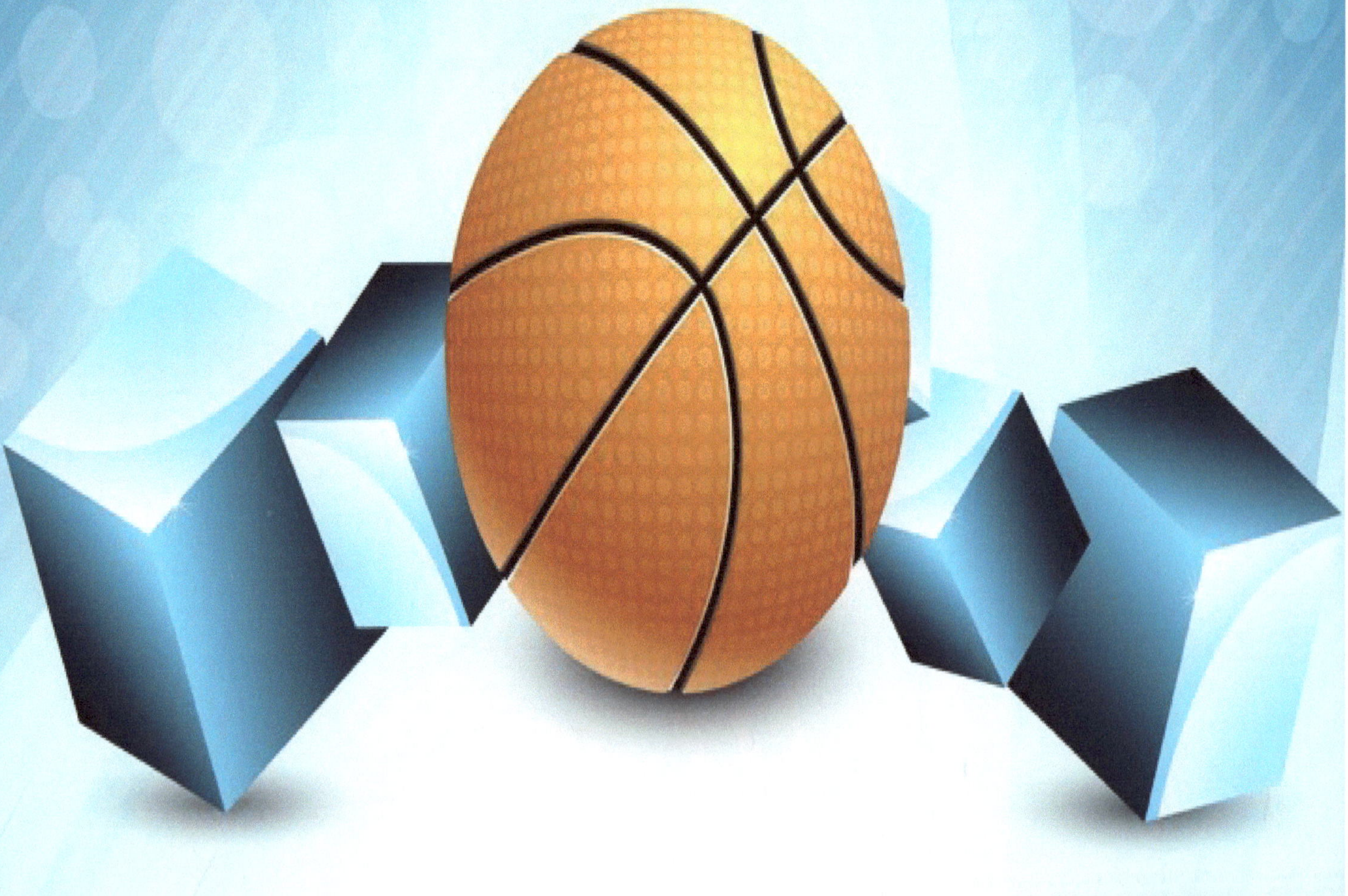

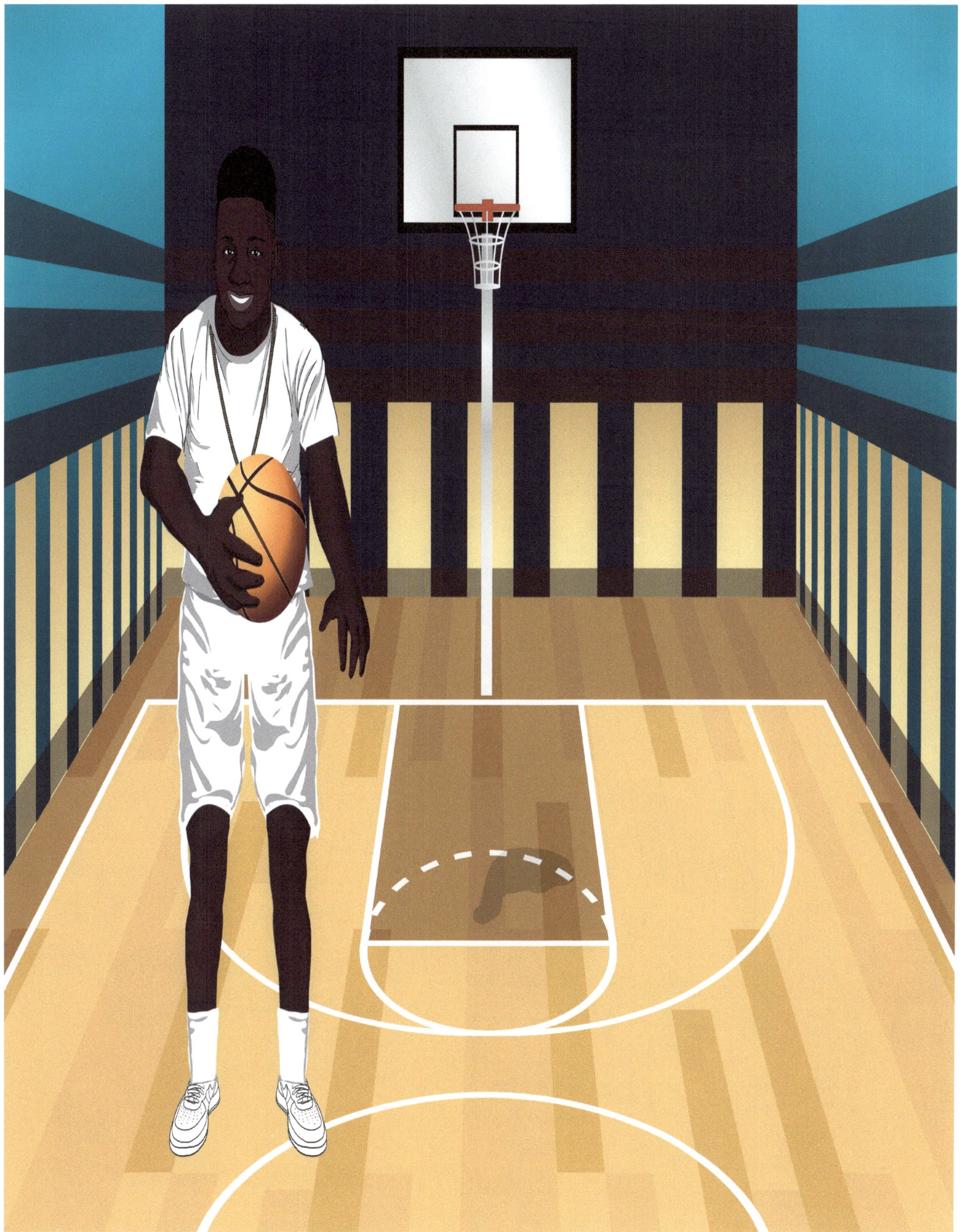

The coach was walking around the room with a box of uniforms. He asked all the young men to put on the shorts and jersey. Ricky began to sweat out of fear. He didn't want the other students to see his legs.

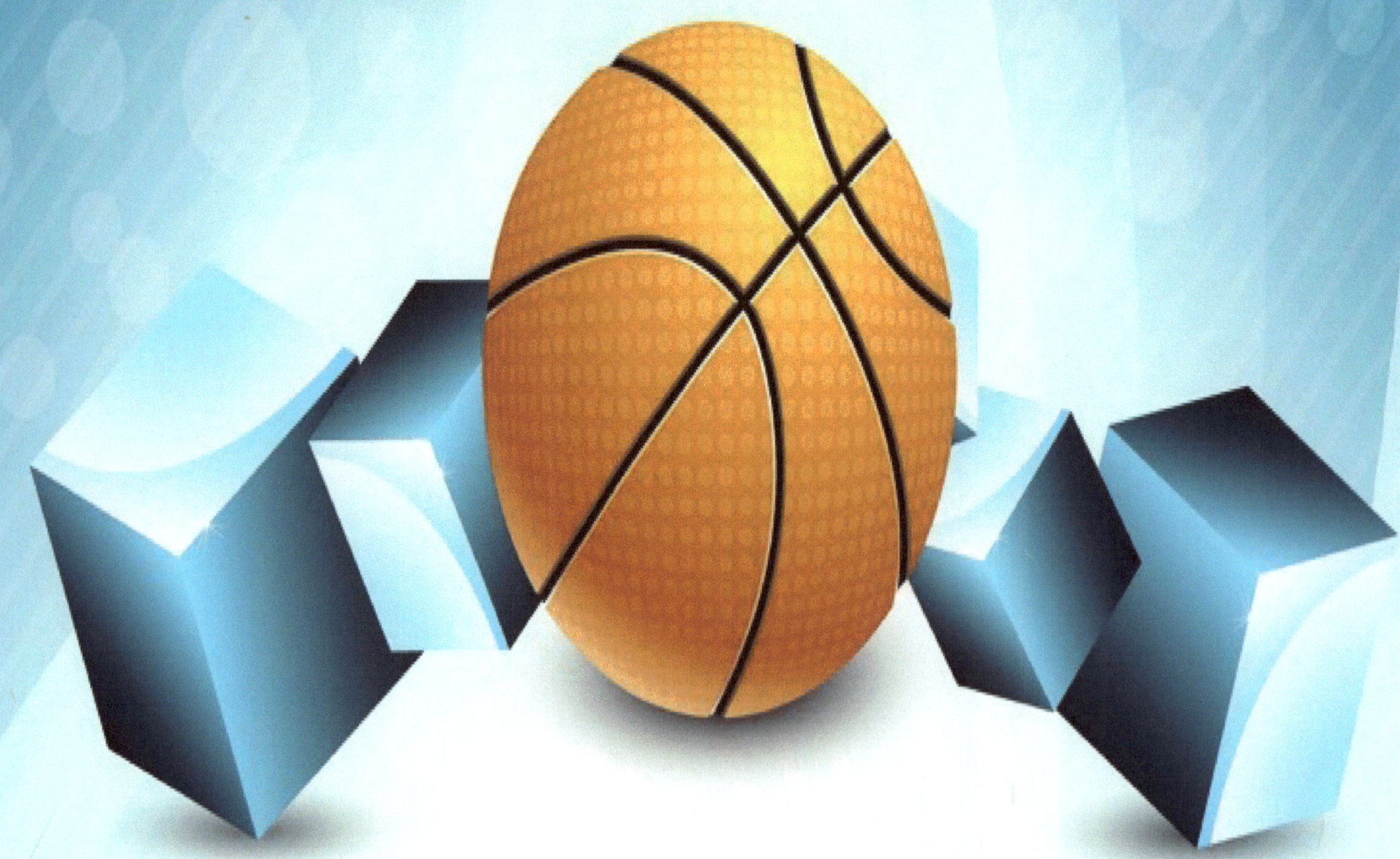

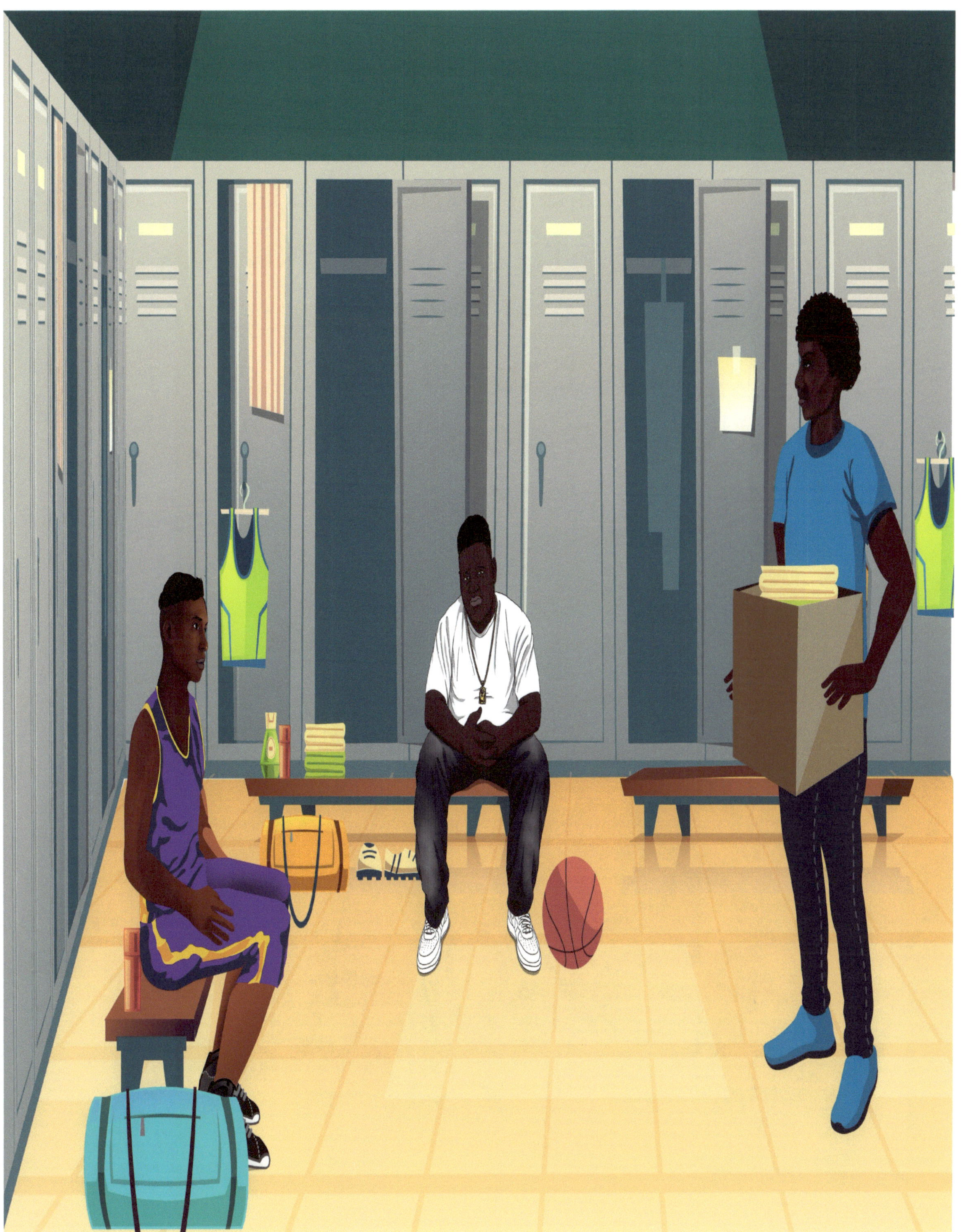

Rickey suffers from severe Atopic dermatitis also known as eczema. The students are always teasing him about it. He has tried everything to clear up his skin, but nothing works.

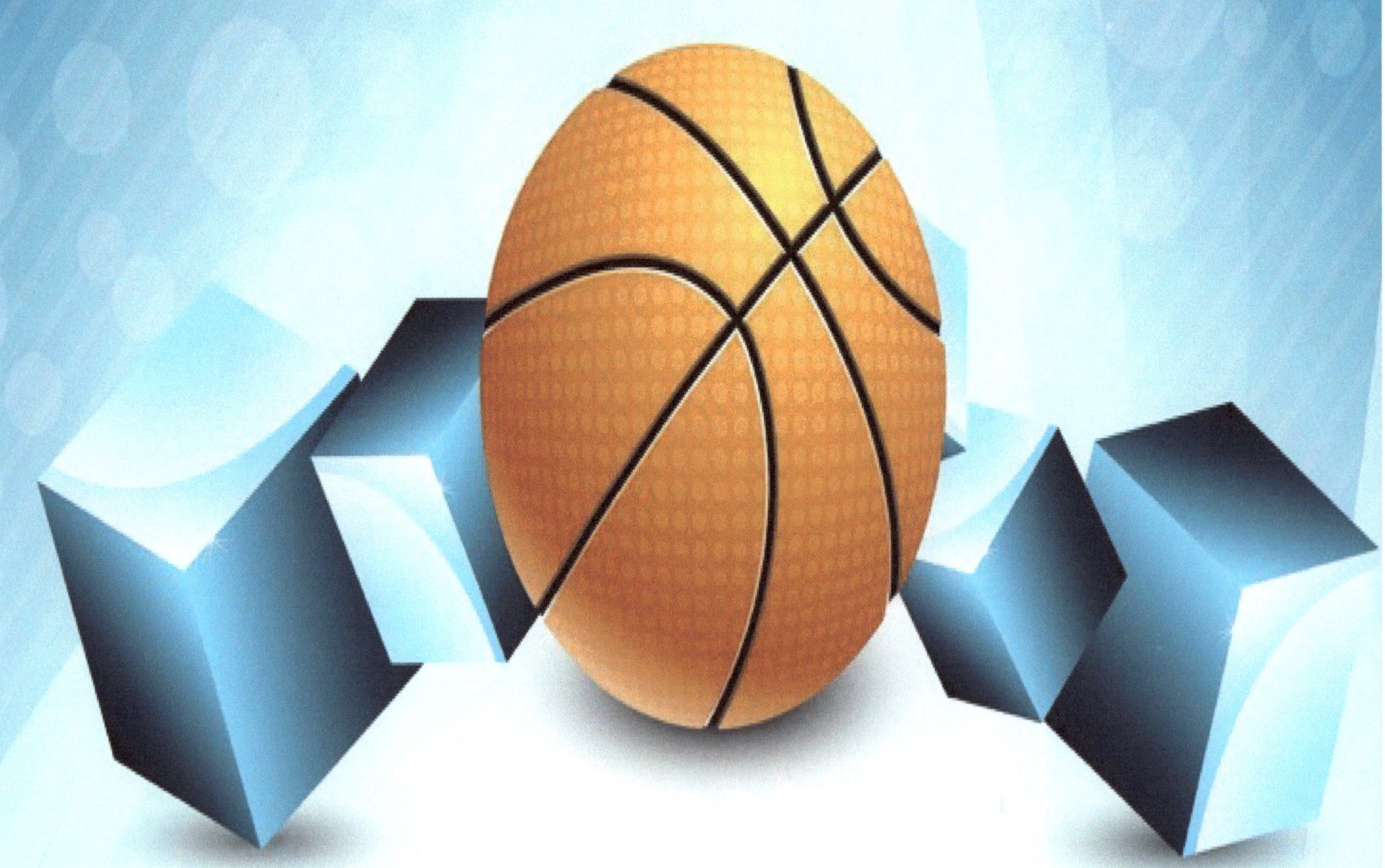

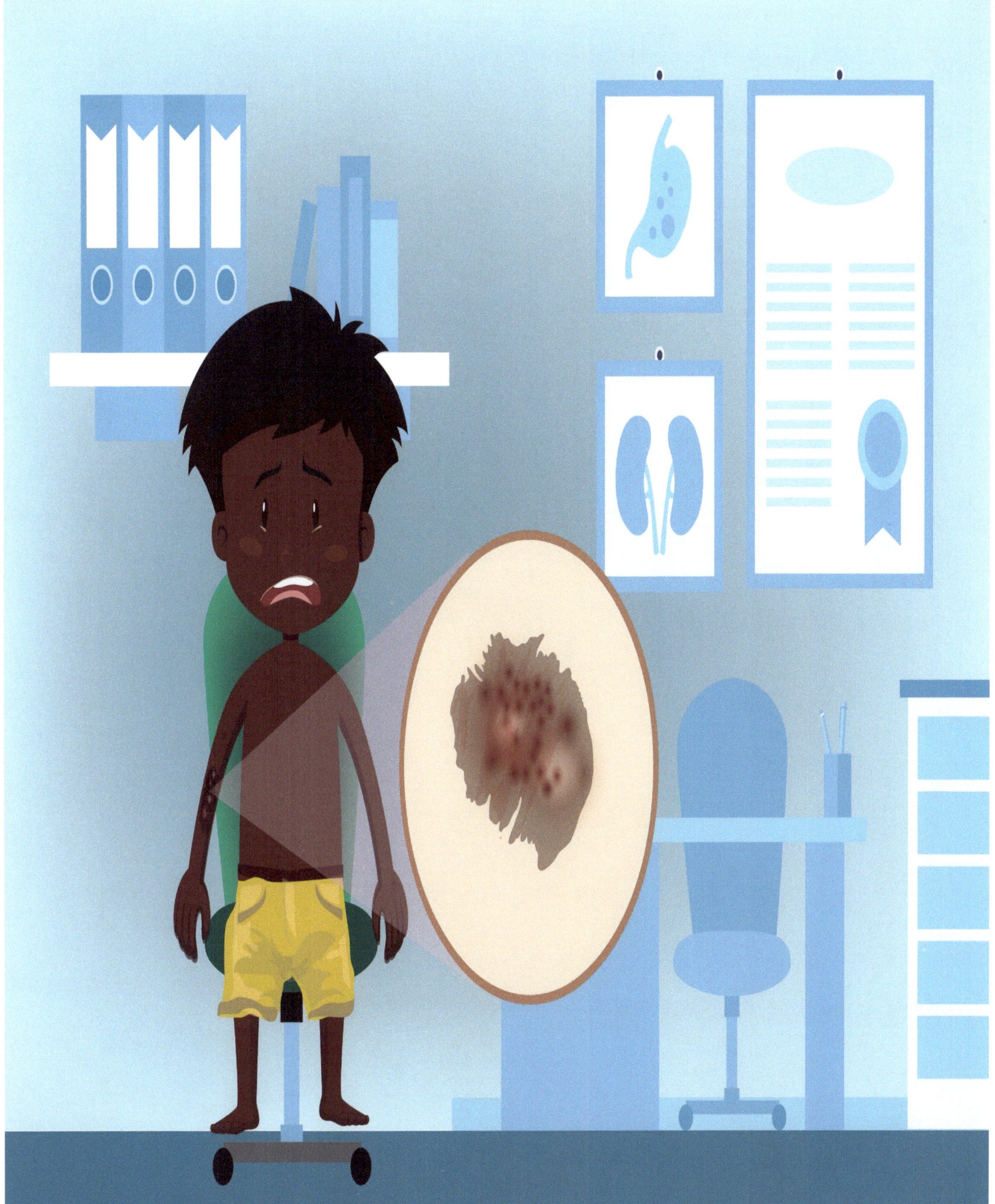

As the coach is approaching Ricky, Ricky runs out and says he must go. Ricky ran all the way home. When he walked in the door, his mother asked how was try outs. Ricky began to cry.

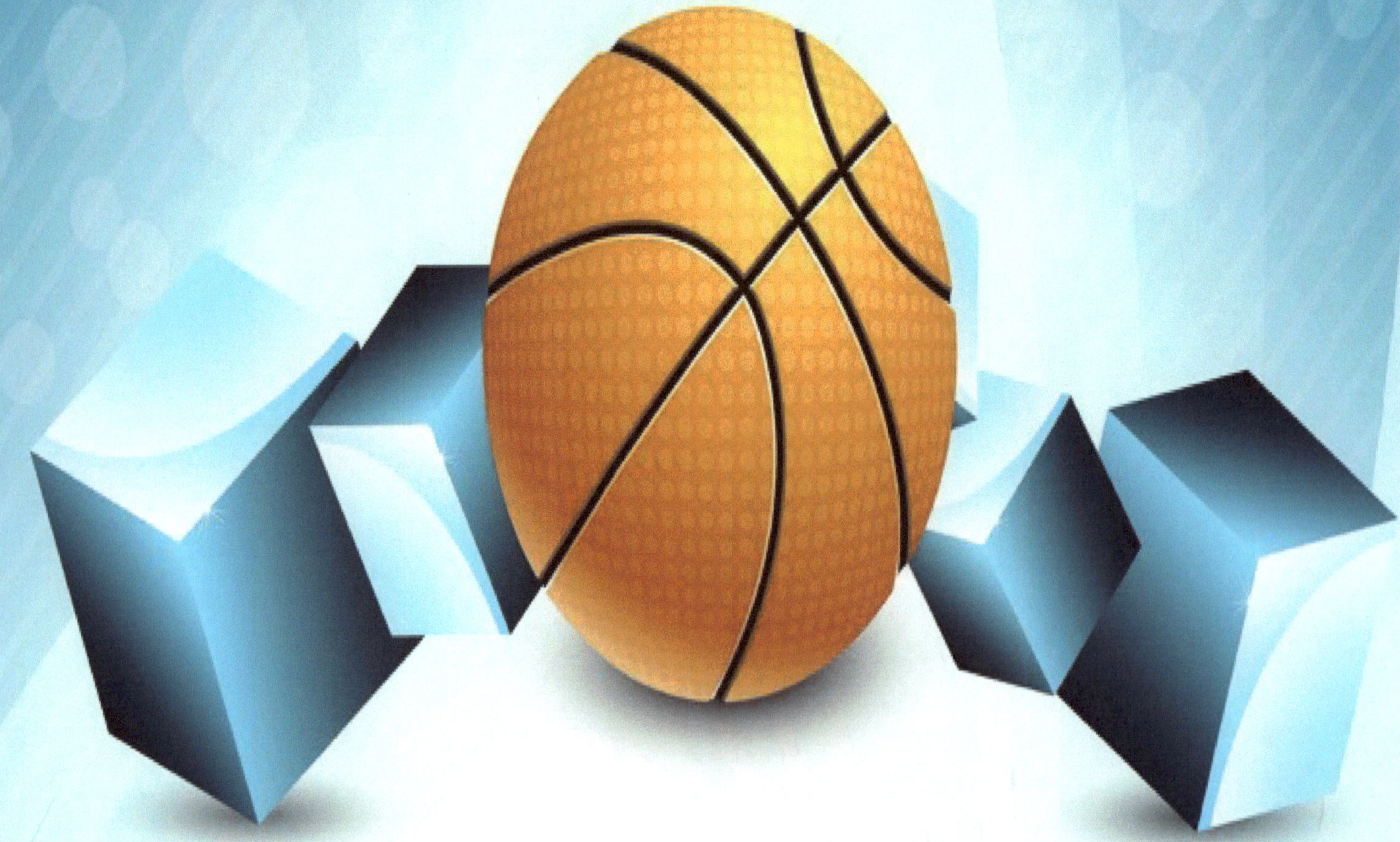

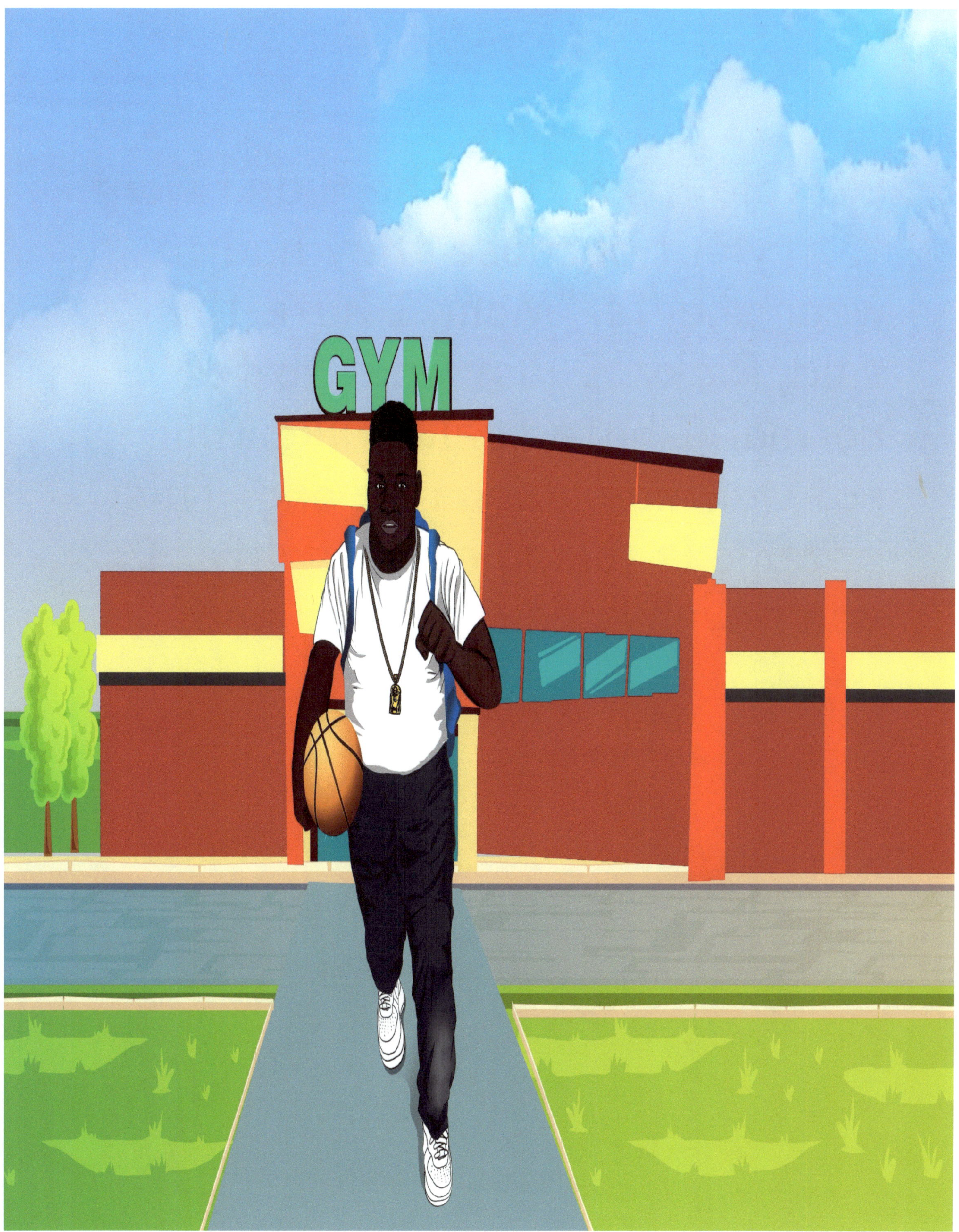

GYM

He told his mother he didn't want to try out because they had to wear shorts. "Mom, I hate this!" said, Ricky. I just want to feel normal. I hate feeling like I am not wanted or don't belong. This eczema is taking over my life, I don't even have a best friend.

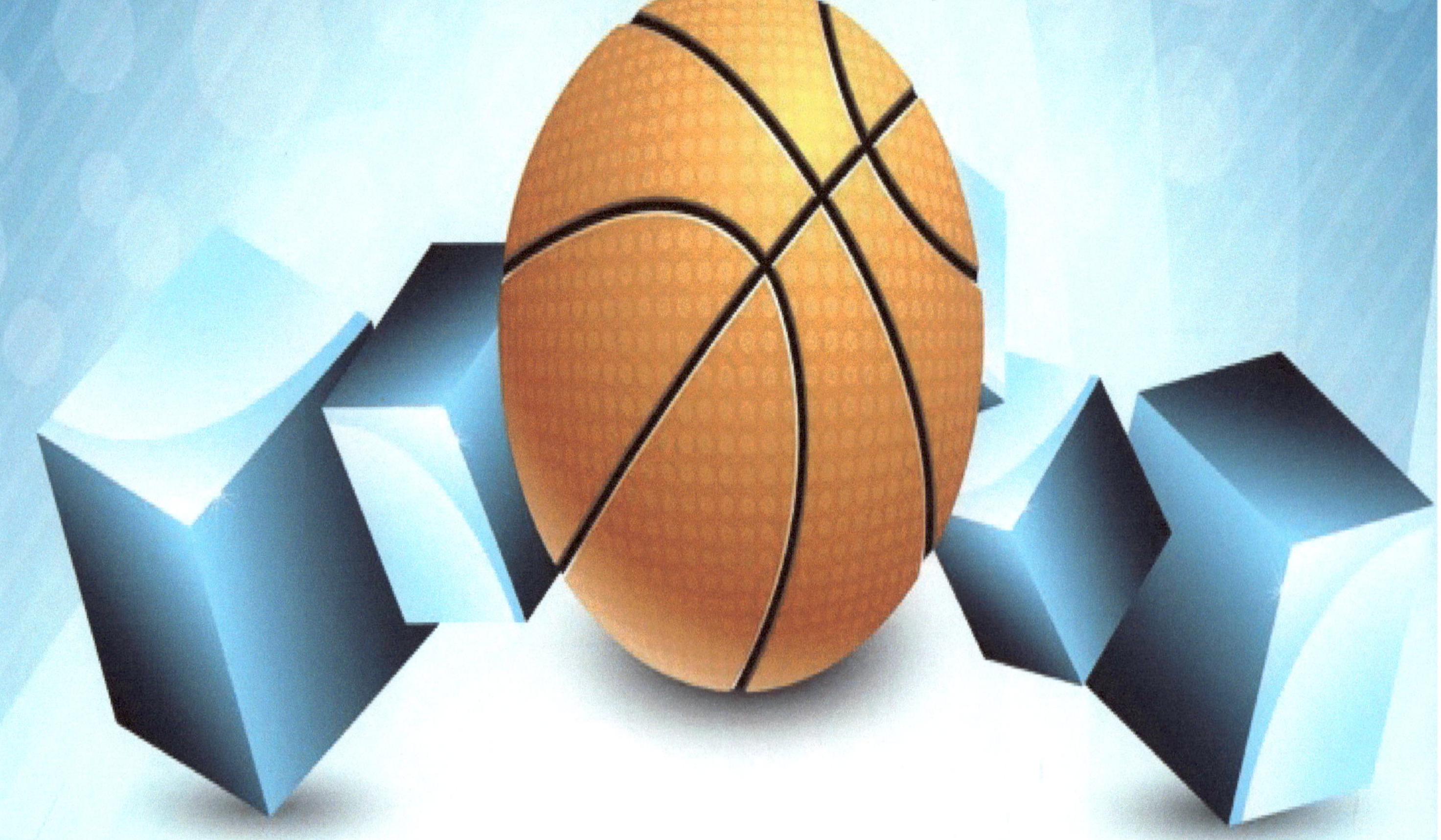

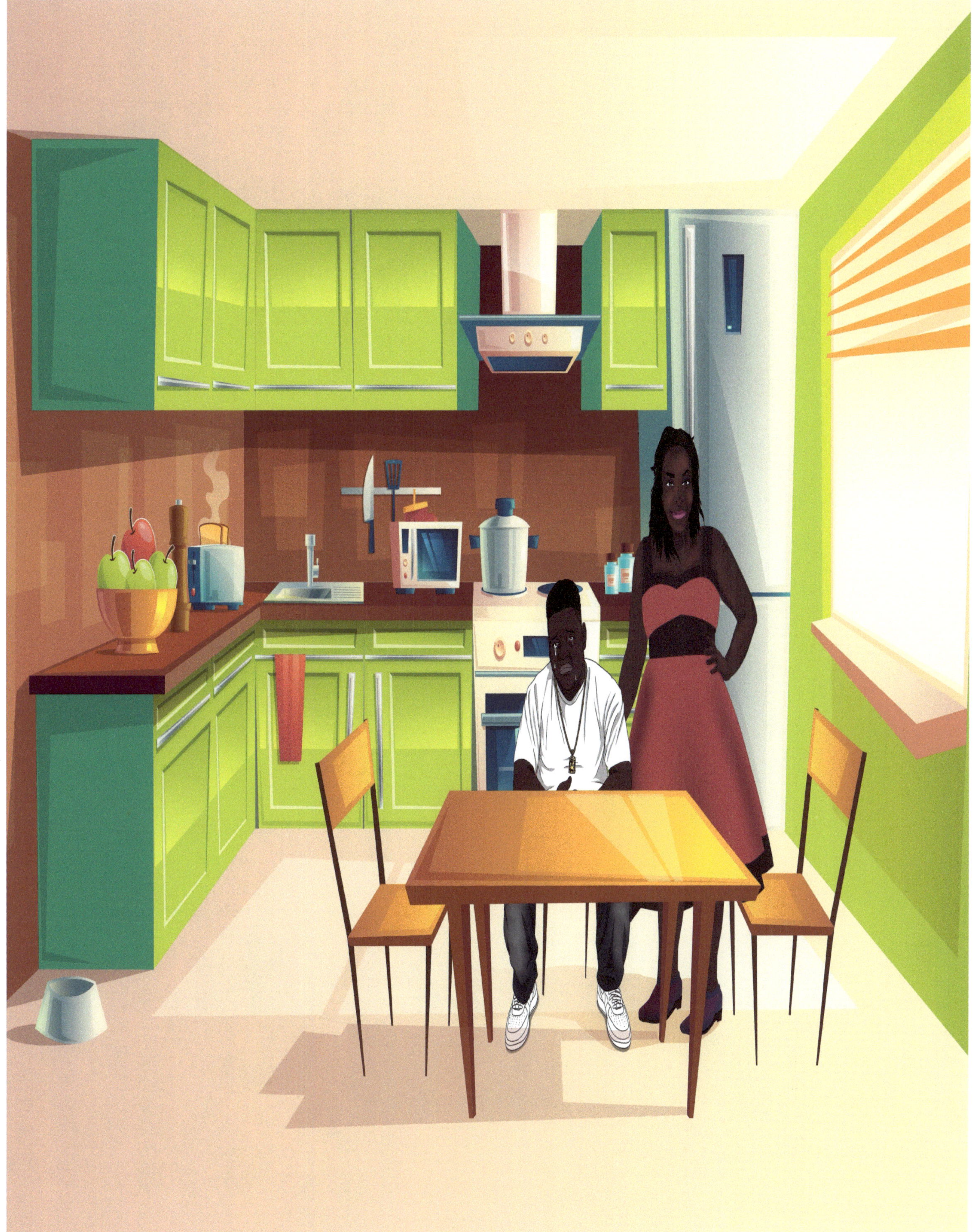

Ricky's mother reminded him of how amazing, funny, handsome, stylish and talented he is. "You can't worry about what others may say to you or about you. You are not here for them.

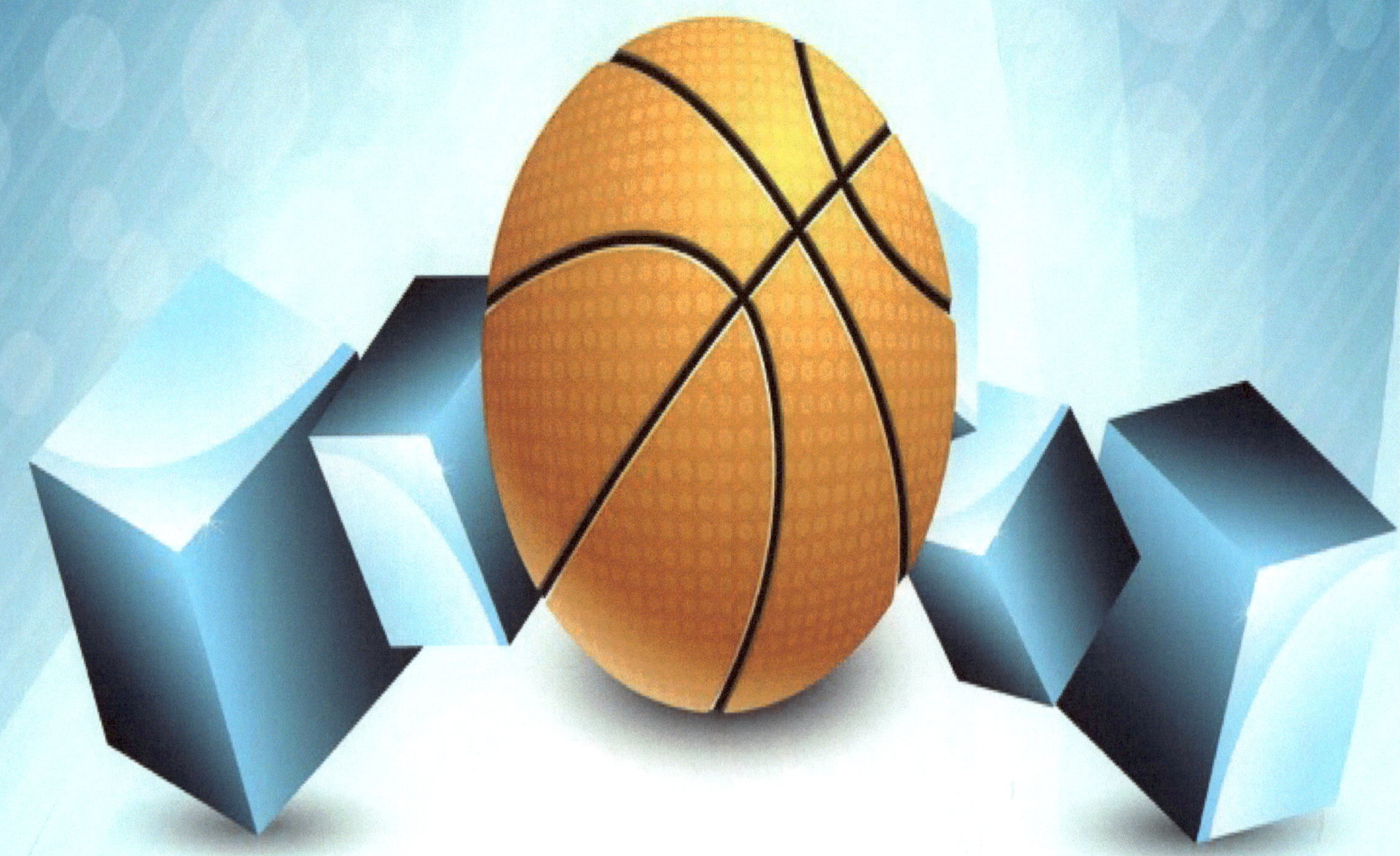

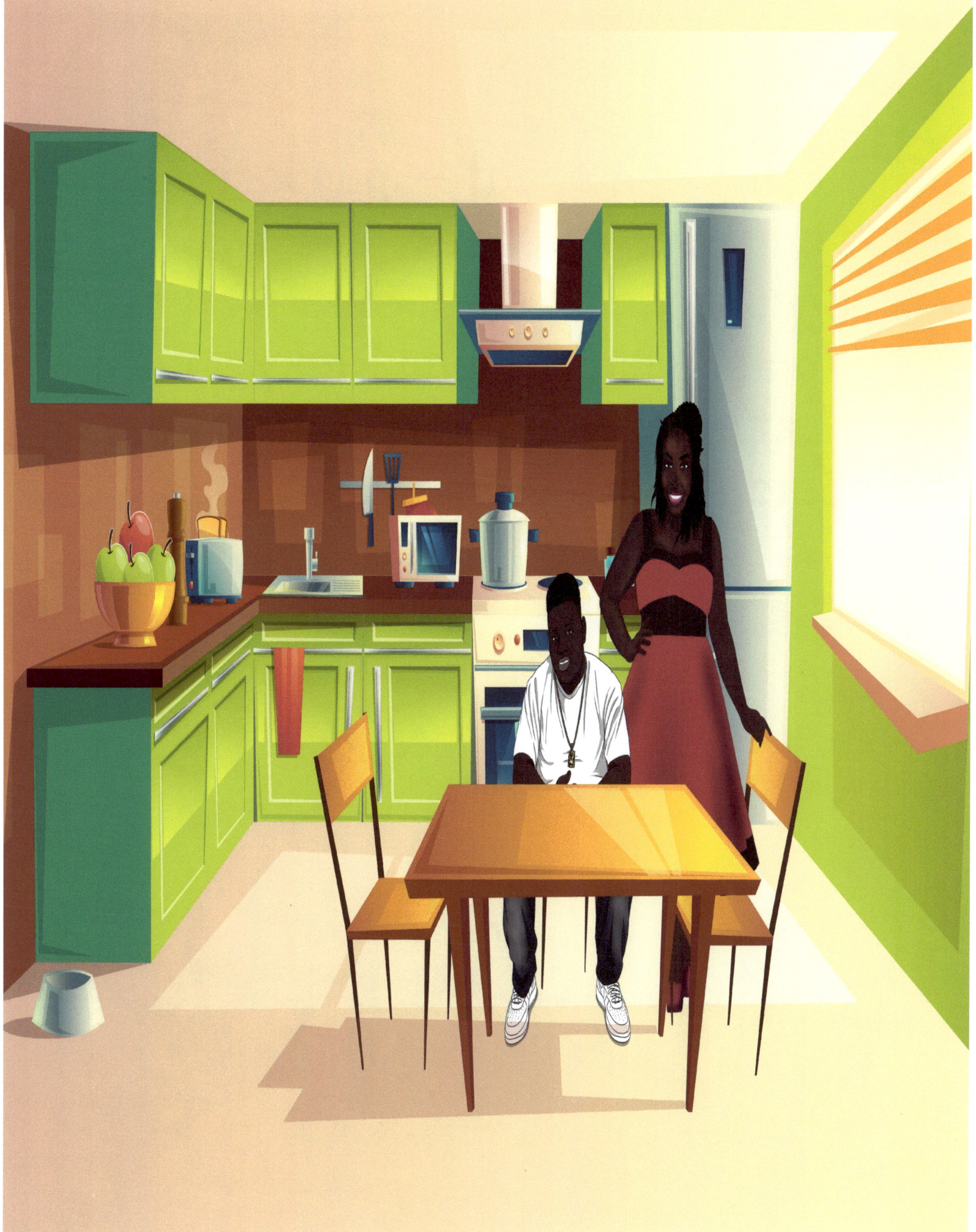

There is a greater purpose on your life. You need to stay encouraged." said Ricky's mom. You are right mom! Ricky said. "Let's get you back to tryouts!" Said Ricky's mom.

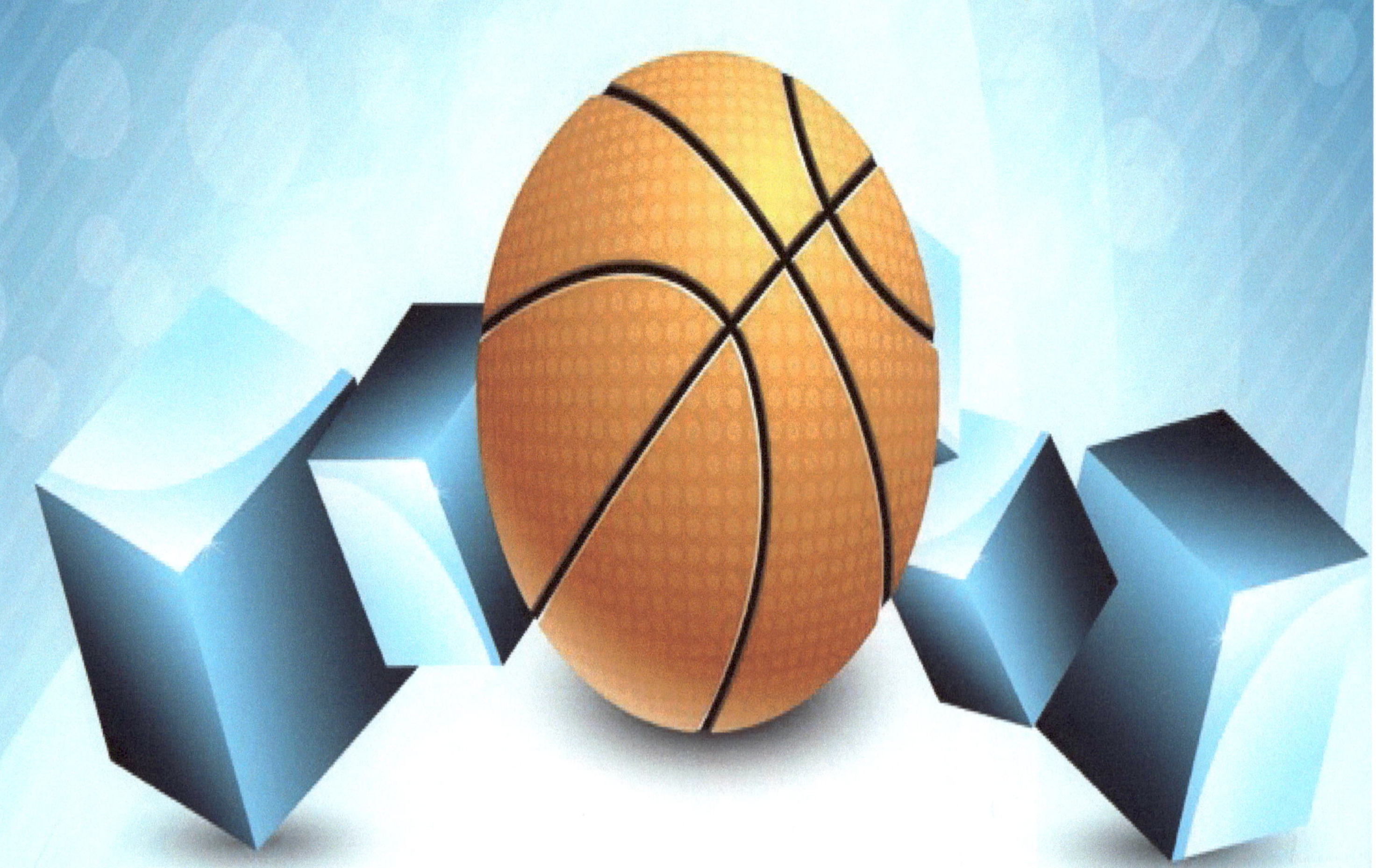

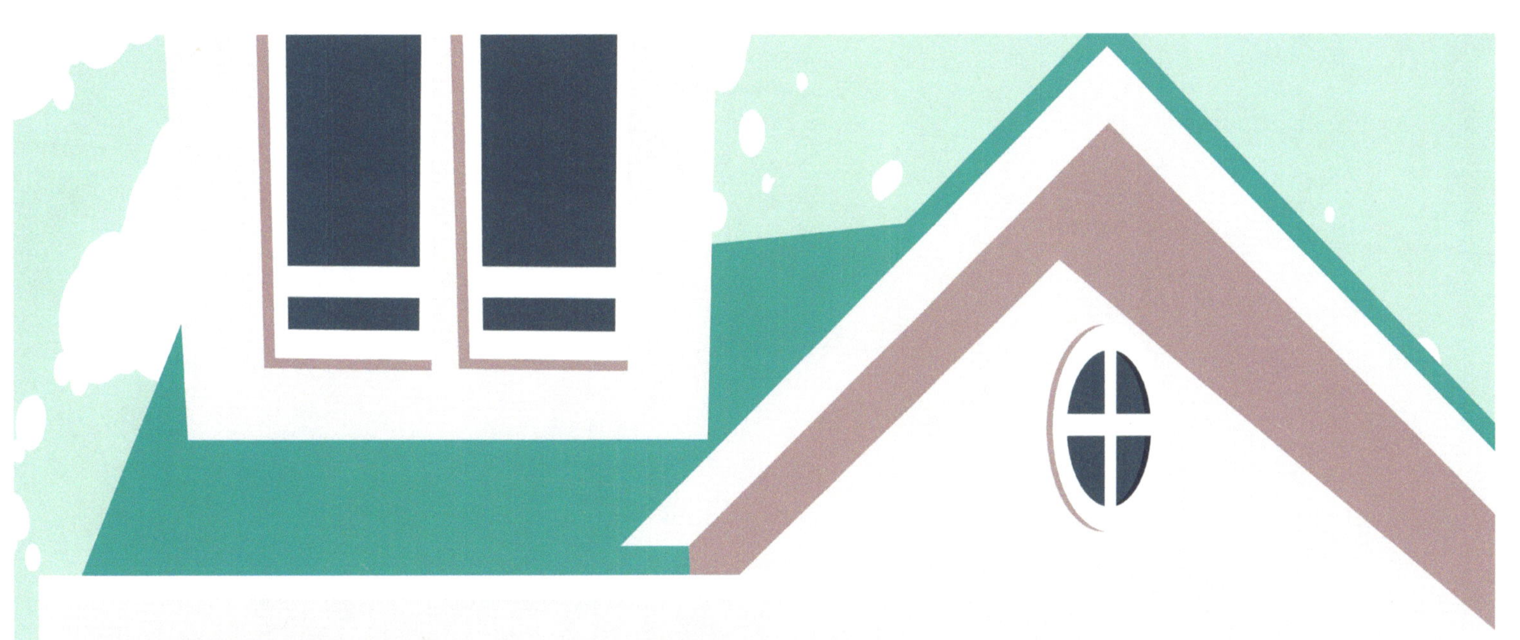
RICKY
HOUSE

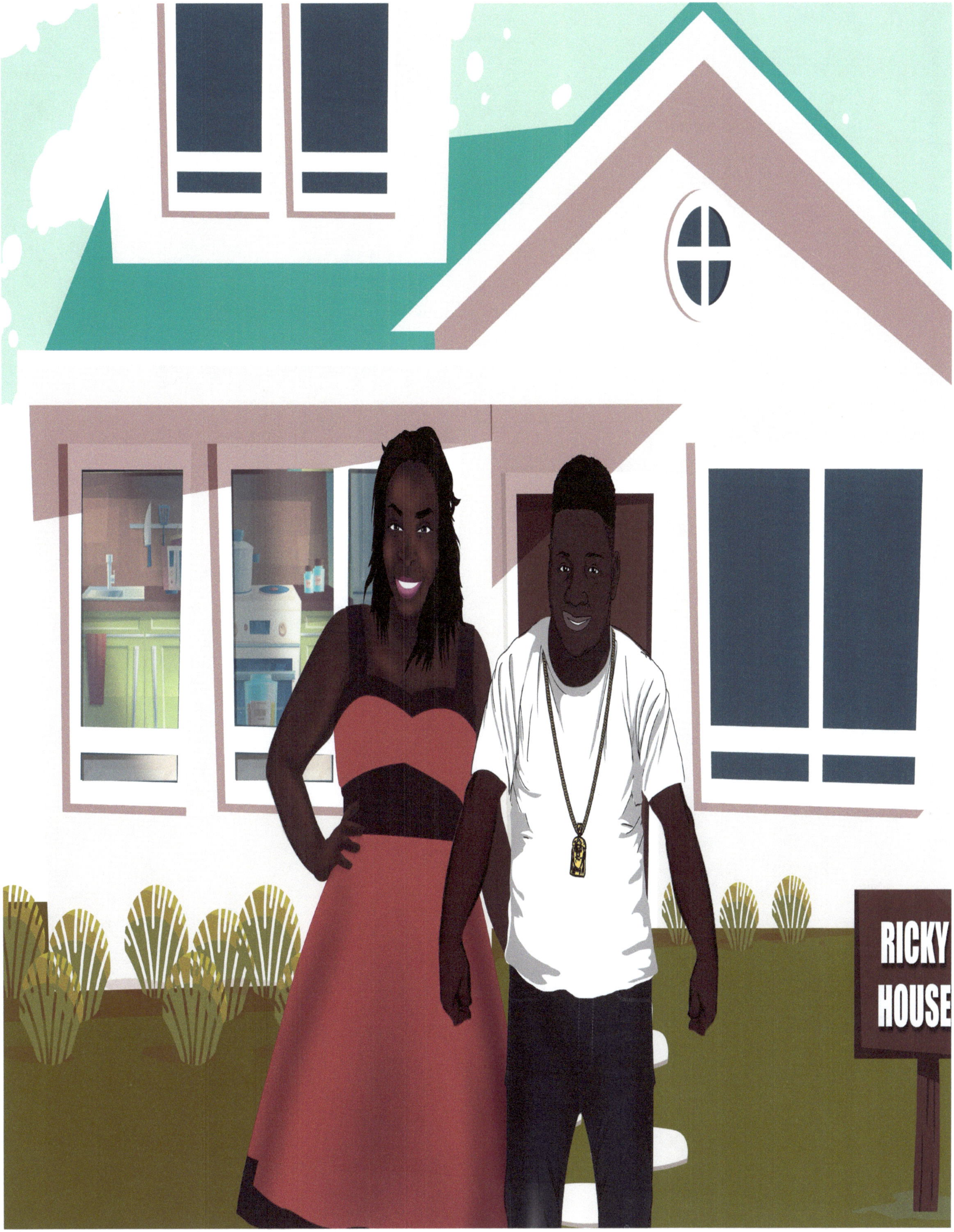

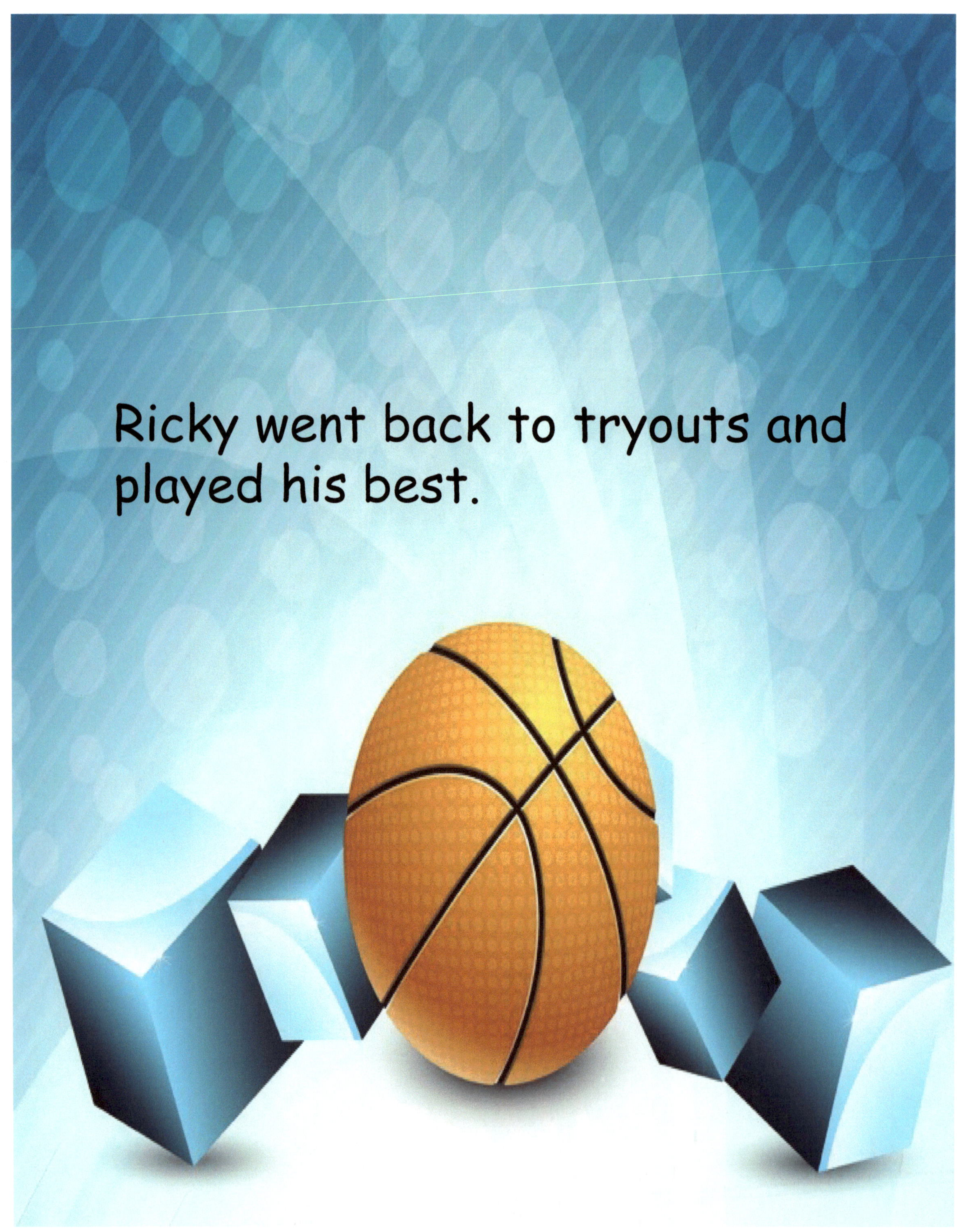

Ricky went back to tryouts and played his best.

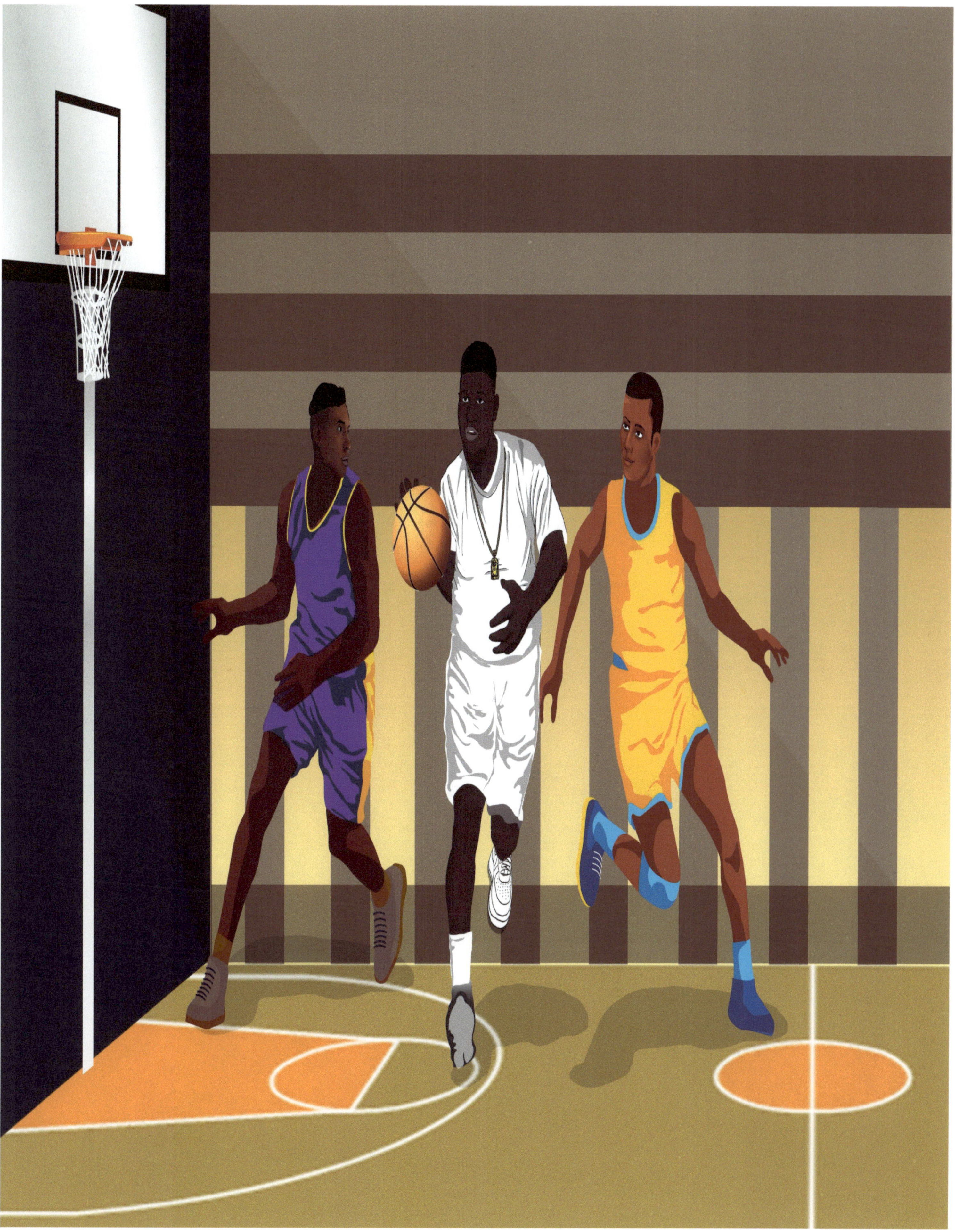

After tryouts, Ricky came home, and his Grandma was there waiting. He told her he made the team and is the starting point guard. His Grandmother said," Just like I knew you would." Ricky no longer let his eczema take over his life, instead he took over his eczema.

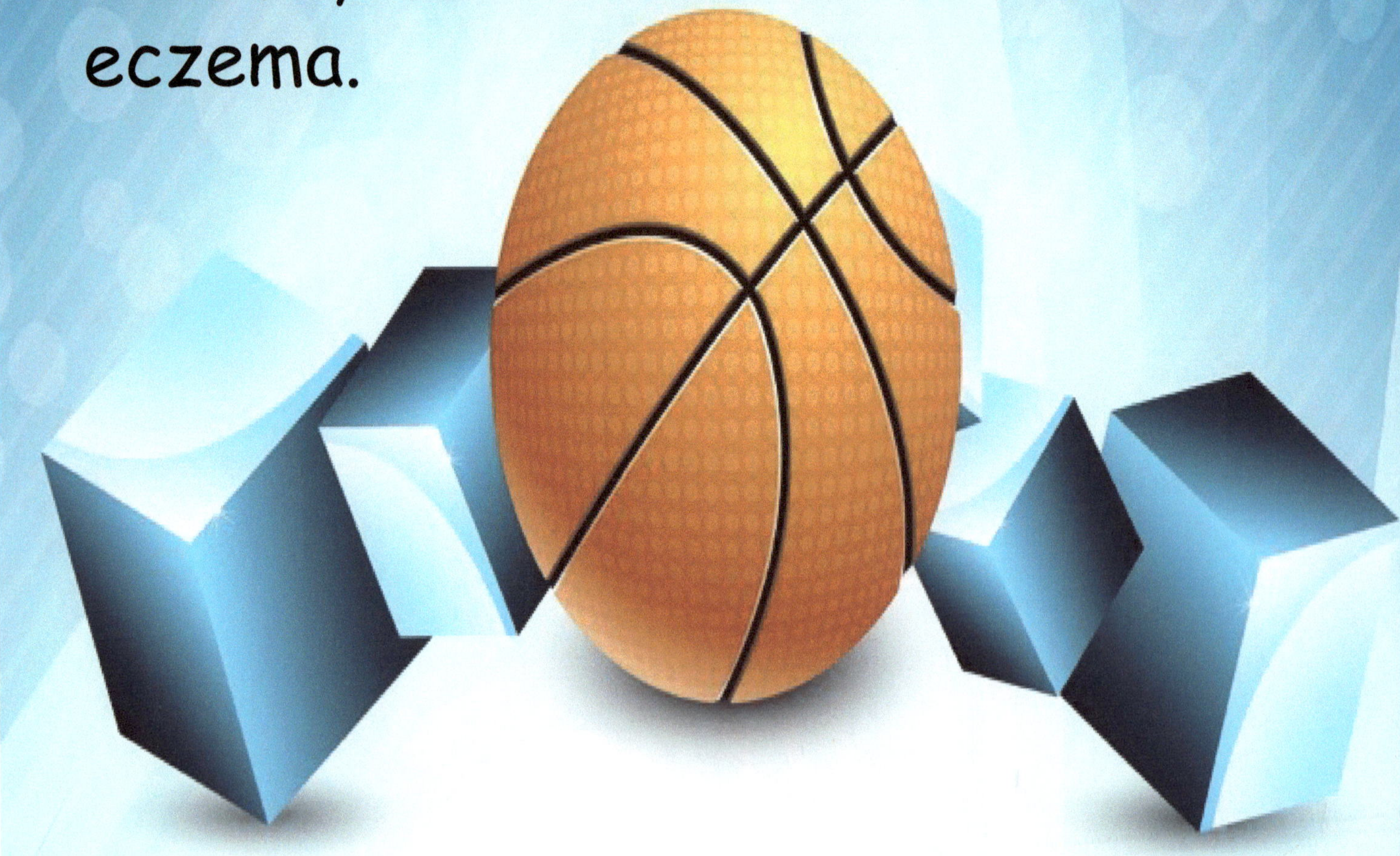

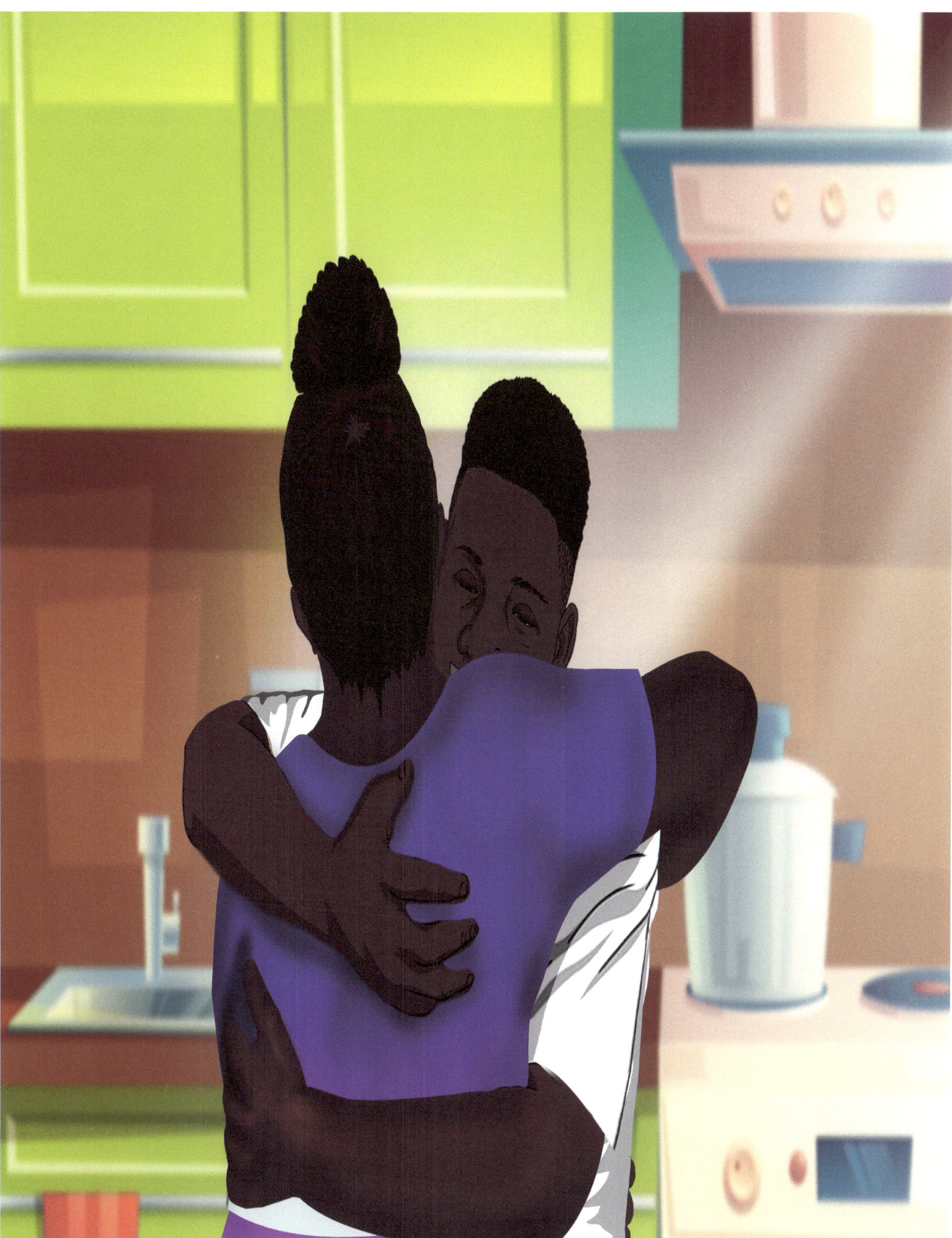

<u>*DEDICATION*</u>

I would like to dedicate this book to my Grandmother Frazier, and my Mother. I love you two so much. You two, always make sure that I make it to every single doctor's appointment and always believed in me and supported my dreams. I also must give a BIG THANK YOU to the Dermatology Doctors at Children's Hospital of Wisconsin. From birth, you made sure I received the best possible care and made it a priority to find the right medication for me and my eczema.

Thanks, you all are the real MVP'S!

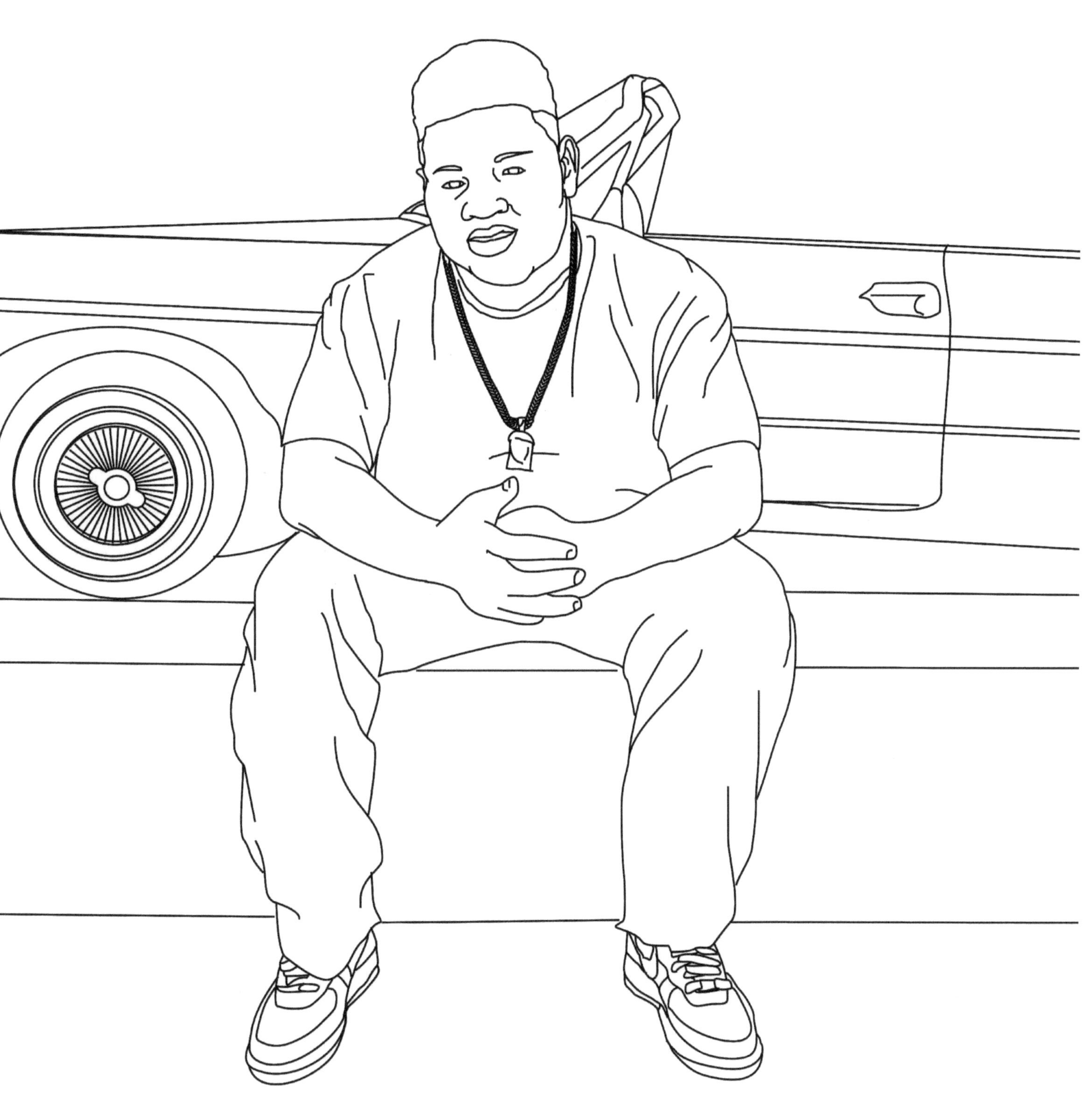

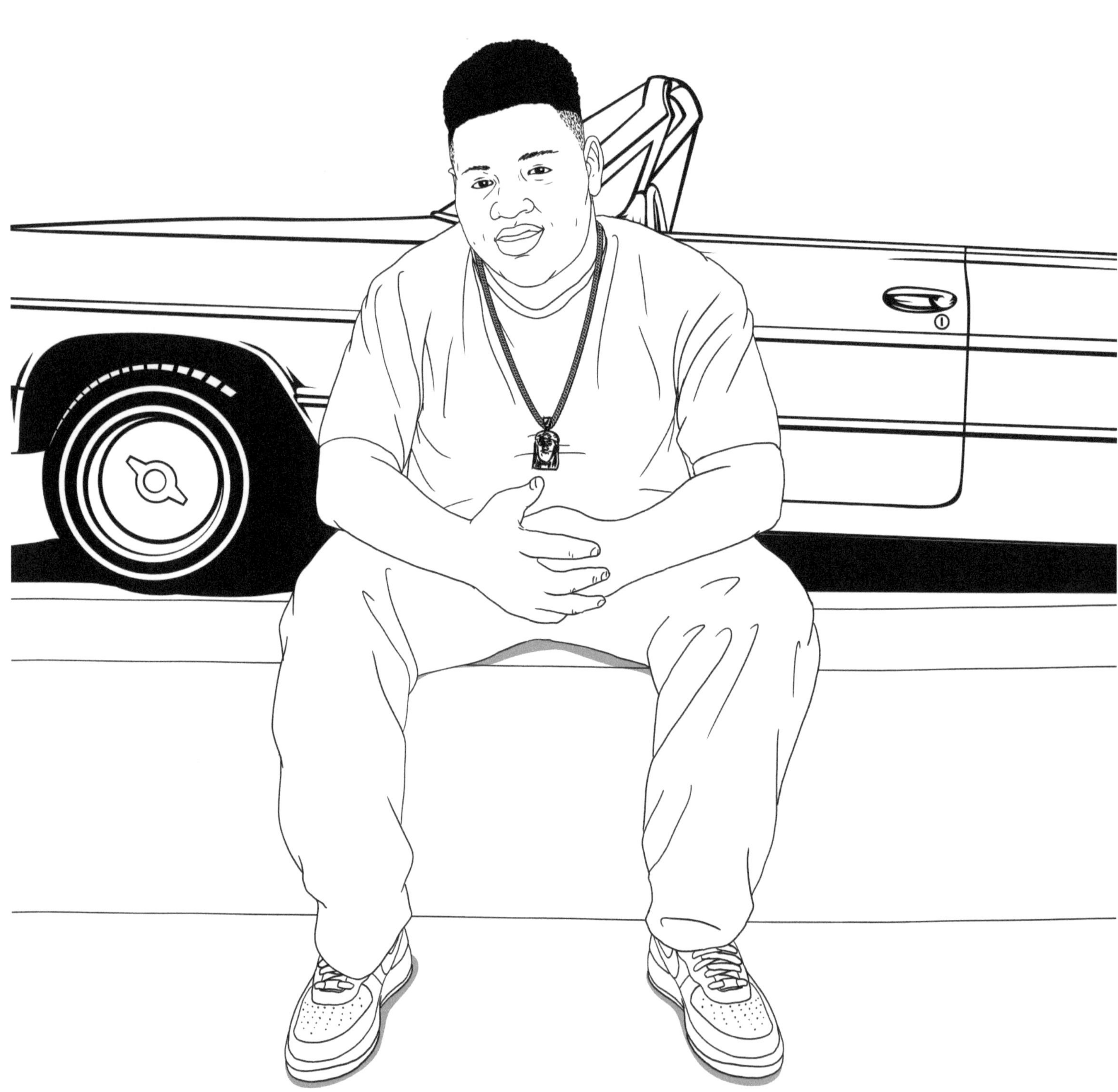